21-Day Sugar Detox Demystified

Drop Sugar to Cut Cravings and Lose Weight

Table of Contents

INTRODUCTION 4

CHAPTER ONE: WHAT IS A SUGAR DETOX? 5

What Does Sugar Do to Your Body? 5

Are You Addicted to Sugar? 6

CHAPTER TWO: BASICS OF THE SUGAR DETOX 8

Principles of the Detox 8

Foods to Eat/Avoid 9

CHAPTER THREE: SUGAR DETOX RECIPES 13

Breakfast Recipes 13

    Banana Almond Smoothie 14

    Glowing Greens Smoothie 15

    Vanilla Coconut Smoothie 16

    3-Ingredient Banana Pancakes 17

    Spiced Pumpkin Pancakes 18

    Easy Almond Flour Muffins 19

    Tomato Basil Omelet 20

    Mushroom Scallion Omelet 21

Lunch Recipes 22

    Cream of Cauliflower Soup 23

    Chilled Avocado Soup 24

    Creamy Curried Carrot Soup 25

    Hearty Chicken Vegetable Soup 26

    Avocado Kale Salad with Almonds 28

    Warm Quinoa Vegetable Salad 29

    Spring Salad with Balsamic Dressing 31

    Chilled Three-Bean Salad 32

Dinner Recipes 33

    Rosemary Roasted Chicken Legs 34

    Coconut-Crusted Baked Halibut 35

    Balsamic-Glazed Pork Chops 36

    Bacon-Wrapped Scallops 37

Slow-Cooker Beef Stew 38

Chicken and Vegetable Curry 40

Baked Haddock with Fresh Salsa 42

Spicy Seafood Soup 43

Snack Recipes **44**

Crispy Kale Chips 45

Cinnamon Baked Banana Chips 46

Sweet and Salty Trail Mix 47

Spicy Mixed Nuts 48

Avocado Chocolate Mousse 49

Baked Apples with Walnuts 50

Mini Banana Nut Muffins 51

Roasted Cauliflower Bites 52

CHAPTER FOUR: AFTER YOU DETOX 53

CONCLUSION 54

REFERENCES .... ERROR! BOOKMARK NOT DEFINED.

Introduction

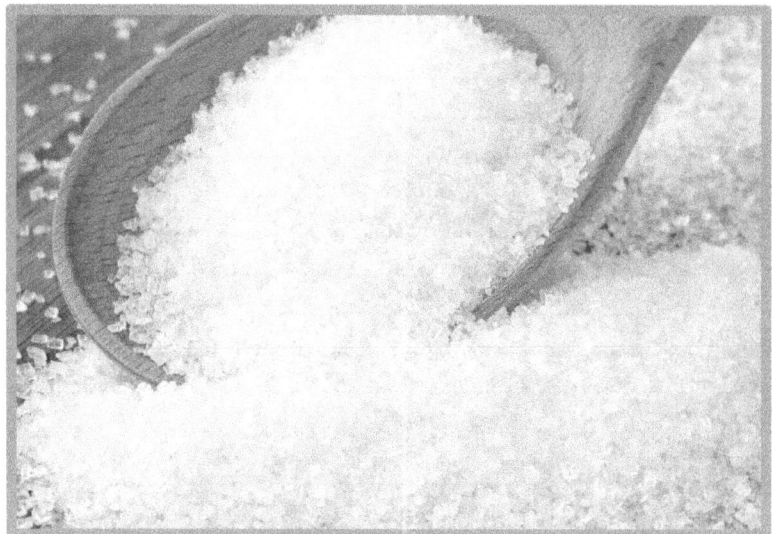

If you pay attention to popular health and fitness trends, you are probably at least a little familiar with the sugar detox. Even if you haven't heard of it, however, the concept is pretty simple – you give up all forms of sugar for 21 days straight. This may seem a little extreme, especially if you are used to eating a lot of sugar, but it can have some significant benefits for your health and wellbeing. Numerous studies have shown that the overconsumption of sugar leads to a variety of serious health problems – not only does it contribute to Type 2 Diabetes but it can also increase your risk for cardiac problems and certain types of cancer. If you are serious about improving your health and kicking your sugar addiction, the 21-day sugar detox may be the way to go.

Though the idea of giving up sugar may seem extreme, or even unimaginable to you, it may actually be easier than you think. This book will guide you through the basics of the sugar detox to help you understand what it is and why it is necessary – you may be shocked to learn about the dangerous effects sugar can have on your body. After you learn the basics about the detox you will receive some tips for making changes to your diet to remove all forms of sugar (including artificial sweeteners). Once you are ready to start your detox you will find a collection of delicious sugar-free recipes for breakfast, lunch, dinner and snacks to help you make it through your 21 days. Finally, once you complete your detox, you will find some helpful tips for slowly incorporating natural sugars back into your diet.

Chapter One: What is a Sugar Detox?

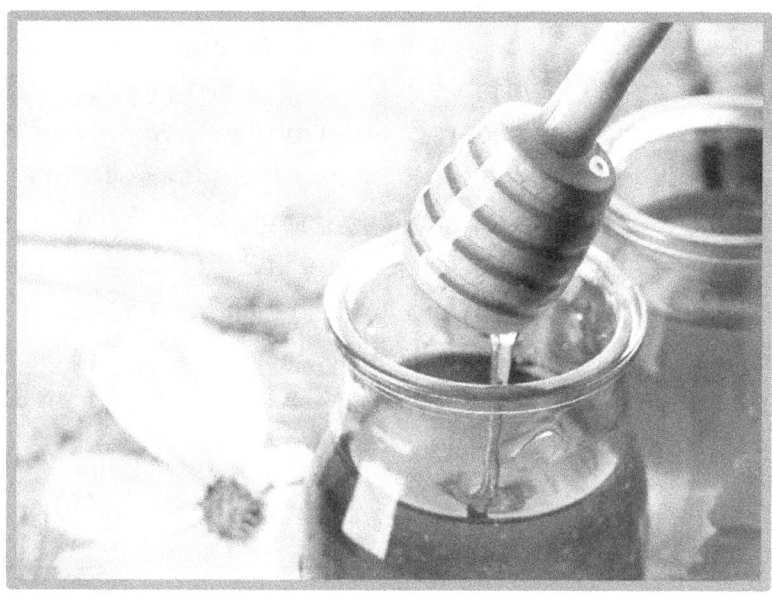

In the simplest terms, a sugar detox is a period during which you consume no sugar of any form – this includes natural sweeteners, artificial sweeteners and refined sugars. There are many reasons for which a person might engage in a sugar detox but the most common is to kick sugar cravings and to break an addiction to sugar. You may not realize it, but the average American consumes over 150 pounds of refined sugar each year – that equates to more than 6 cups in a single week! It is unlikely that you eat a whole cup of a sugar at a time, but you may not realize just how much is added to the foods you eat regularly or how quickly a little bit of sugar a few times a day can add up over the course of a week.

What Does Sugar Do to Your Body?

Sugar consumption can wreak havoc on your body, often in ways you do not realize. The most obvious danger of consuming too much sugar, however, is the extra calories. In a study conducted by the U.S. Department of Health and Human Services, it was revealed that the average American man consumes an extra 335 calories per day from added sugar alone – for women, that number was around 240. These calories are on top of your daily recommended calorie intake which can lead to a significant surplus of calories throughout the week. Even a surplus of 250 calories per day can add up to an extra 1,750 calories per week – for some people that is an entire day's worth of calories!

The role that sugar plays in the body is fairly complicated because different types of sugar have different effects. Glucose is the most common type of sugar and it serves as the body's primary source of available energy – it is metabolized quickly rather than being stored. When you consume sugar, it is transported through your blood to the pancreas where it stimulates the production of insulin. That insulin, in turn, travels to your brain and triggers the release of certain chemicals which tell your body that you are full and it is time to stop eating. Fructose, a different type of sugar, is metabolized by the body in a different way – your body still produces insulin but this type of sugar contains a protein called leptin which inhibits your brain's ability to recognize the fact that you are full. As a result, you may continue eating past the point where you should no longer be hungry – this is where those extra calories come from.

In addition to these chemical effects of sugar on the body, the consumption of sugar can lead to other dangerous effects. <u>Some of these effects are listed below</u>:

- Some sugars cause a "sugar high" followed by a severe crash
- Sugar consumption can lead to spikes in blood glucose levels which leads to inflammation – inflammation can increase the effects of aging on your skin
- Eating too much sugar may impact your endocrine system, the system responsible for your hormones, which can lead to hormone imbalance
- Overconsumption of fructose can lead to memory problems
- Digested sugars may bond to collagen in your skin cells which may make conditions like acne and rosacea worsen
- Eating too much sugar can lead to digestive disorders and may also cause symptoms including bloating and gas

Are You Addicted to Sugar?

Now that you know the basics about how sugar impacts your body and how dangerous it can be, you may be curious to know how much your own sugar consumption puts you at risk for these negative impacts. Below you will find a series of questions to ask yourself to help you assess how much sugar you really consume on a daily basis and whether or not you may be addicted. The results of this quiz may surprise you and may also help lead you to a decision regarding whether a sugar detox is the right choice for you.

1. Do you regularly consume candy and sweet treats?

2. Do you often add sugar or artificial sweeteners to beverages like coffee and tea?

3. Do you suffer from frequent cravings for sugary foods?

4. Do you often find that once you start eating something sugary, you can't stop?

5. Do you find yourself eating more of sugary foods than you normally would of other kinds of foods without feeling full?

6. Do you often have trouble getting out of bed in the morning?

7. Do you require caffeine, chocolate, or other substances to keep you awake during the day?

8. Do you eat something sweet with or after most of your meals?

If you answered "Yes" to even one of these questions, you have probably experienced the effects of sugar on your body. Answering "Yes" to three or more questions indicates a likely addiction to sugar which means that engaging in a sugar detox would be highly beneficial for you.

Chapter Two: Basics of the Sugar Detox

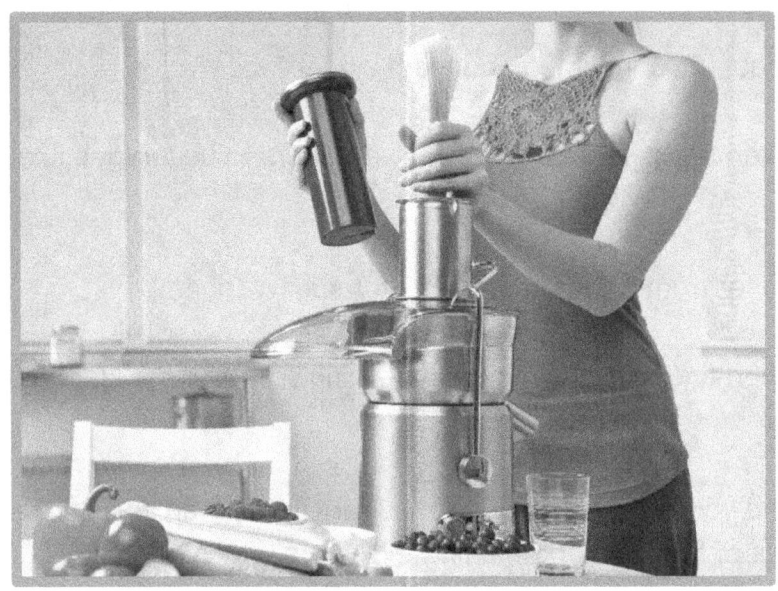

Now that you know the basics about what a sugar detox is and how it can benefit you, you are ready to get into some of the details. In order to reap the maximum benefit from a sugar detox, it is recommended that you follow the detox for 21 days – three weeks. You can go shorter if you must, and going longer is always an option as well. Some people choose to never reincorporate sugar into their diet after finishing the detox – you have that option too. In this chapter you will receive details about what you can and cannot eat on the sugar detox as well as some helpful tips for making the transition from your current diet.

Principles of the Detox

The main principle of the sugar detox is, of course, to cut out all types of sugar – this includes refined sugar, natural sweeteners and artificial sweeteners. Even though artificial sweeteners contain no calories, they still cause a similar reaction in your body to regular sugar. In addition to omitting sugar from your diet, it is also recommended that you omit all gluten-containing grains, especially refined flours. The idea of the sugar detox is to get rid of processed, unhealthy foods to give your body a chance to recover from the damage your current diet is likely doing.

It is up to you how extreme you take the principles of the sugar detox. If you are used to following a fairly strict dietary plan, you may also want to consider omitting dairy products, all grains and legumes. If you don't want to follow such a strict plan, stick to gluten-free grains and limited amounts of legumes and starchy vegetables. If you choose to consume dairy while on a sugar detox, it is recommended that you consume only full-fat dairy – that means whole milk (not skim milk), heavy cream (not half-and-half) and full-fat cheese (not reduced-fat or part-skim). In the next section you will find a detailed list of foods to eat and avoid on the sugar detox.

Foods to Eat/Avoid

Below you will find a detailed list of foods that you can eat freely on the sugar detox as well as those that you should avoid or limit your consumption of. Remember, it is your choice whether you want to include gluten-free grains, legumes and full-fat dairy in your sugar detox but all of the foods on the "Avoid" list should not be consumed at any point during your 21-day detox.

Foods to Eat Freely

Meat and Protein

Beef (all cuts)	Lamb	Scallops
Chicken	Shrimp	Fish (all varieties)
Turkey	Crab	Bacon
Duck	Lobster	Deli meat

Dairy and Eggs

Whole milk	Cottage cheese	Full-fat cheese
Heavy cream	Plain yogurt	Kefir
Sour cream	Cream cheese	

Fruits and Vegetables

Artichoke	Cucumber	Radishes
Asparagus	Eggplant	Snow peas
Bell peppers	Kale	Spinach
Broccoli	Leafy greens	Tomato
Brussels sprouts	Leeks	Turnips
Cabbage	Lettuce	Yellow Squash
Carrots	Mushrooms	Zucchini
Cauliflower	Onions	
Celery	Parsnips	

Grains and Legumes

Amaranth	Brown rice	Millet
Arrowroot	Quinoa	Wild rice
Buckwheat	Dried beans	White rice
Chickpeas	Lentils	

Other Staples

Nuts and seeds	Pure extracts	Plain almond milk
Nut and seed flours	Vinegar (all varieties)	Plain coconut milk
Olive oil	Garlic (dried and fresh)	Canned coconut milk
Coconut oil	Ginger (dried and fresh)	Herbal tea
Fresh herbs	Coconut aminos	Coffee
Dried spices	Unsweetened coconut	

Foods to Eat in Moderation

Fruits and Vegetables

Acorn squash	Winter squash	Granny Smith apple
Butternut squash	Spaghetti squash	Grapefruit
Pumpkin	Green-tipped banana	

Other Foods

Coconut water (unsweetened)

Grass-fed butter or ghee

Foods to Avoid

Fruits and Vegetables

All fruits except green-tipped bananas and Granny Smith apples

Sweet potato

Yams

Cassava

Plantains

Soybeans/edamame

Grains

Refined flours	Cookies and cakes	Wheat
Commercial baking mixes	Enriched pasta	Barley
	Cereal and granola	Rye
Bread and pastries		

Oats	Corn	Grits
Couscous	Polenta	

Other Foods

Peanut butter	Alcohol	Oat milk
Cashew butter	Soft drinks	Store-bought condiments
Dried fruits	Fruit juice	
Soy sauce, tamari	Candy	Store-bought salad dressing
Skim milk	Soy milk	

Now that you understand the sugar detox and know what foods you can and cannot eat, you are ready to get started! In the next chapter you will find a collection of delicious breakfast, lunch, dinner and snack recipes to enjoy while you are following the sugar detox.

Chapter Three: Sugar Detox Recipes

Breakfast Recipes

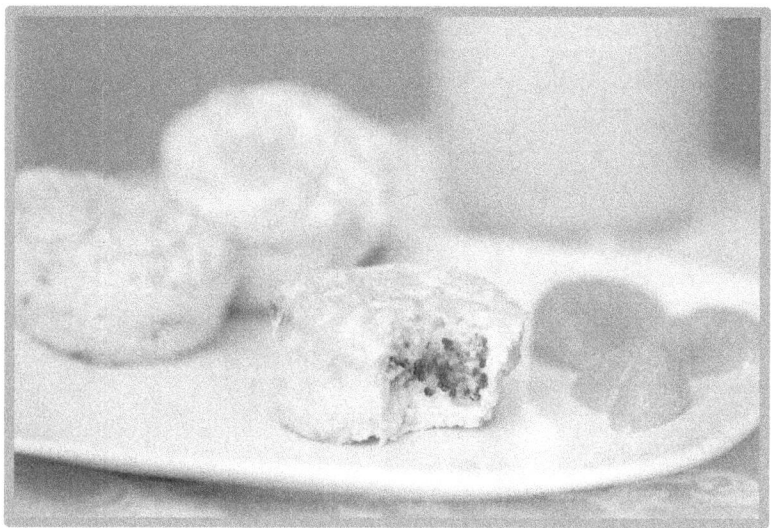

You have probably already heard that breakfast is the most important meal of the day – it gets your metabolism going and provides your body with the fuel it needs to power you through the day. The breakfast recipes you will find in this section are packed with nutrients and flavor – the only thing they are lacking is sugar.

Recipes Included in this Section:

Banana Almond Smoothie

Glowing Greens Smoothie

Vanilla Coconut Smoothie

3-Ingredient Banana Pancakes

Spiced Pumpkin Pancakes

Easy Almond Flour Muffins

Tomato Basil Omelet

Mushroom Scallion Omelet

Banana Almond Smoothie

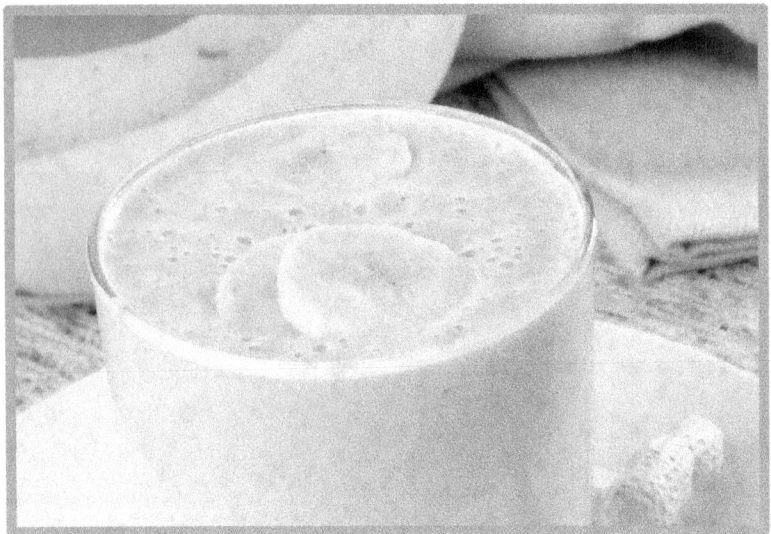

Servings: 2

Ingredients:

- 2 frozen green-tipped bananas, sliced
- 1 cup unsweetened almond milk
- 3 tablespoons raw almonds
- ½ cup ice cubes

Instructions:

1. Combine all ingredients in a blender.
2. Blend on high speed for 30 to 60 seconds until smooth.
3. Pour into glasses and serve immediately.

Glowing Greens Smoothie

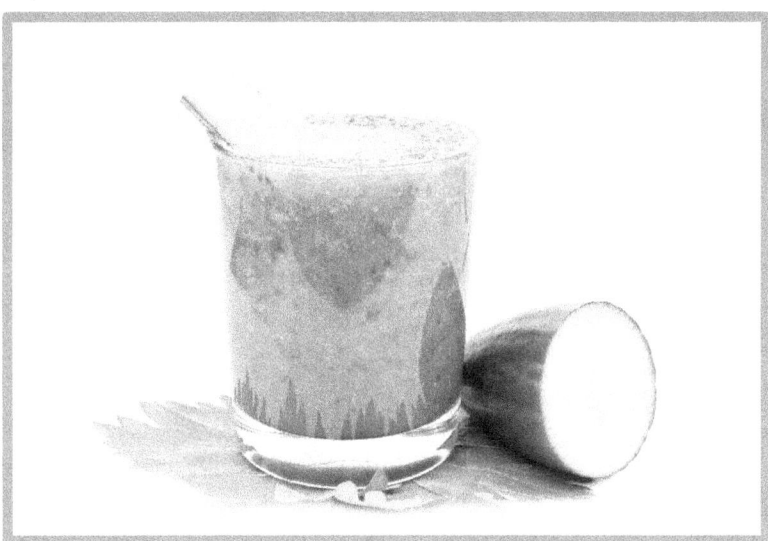

Servings: 2

Ingredients:

- 2 frozen green-tipped bananas, sliced
- 1 cup unsweetened almond milk
- 3 tablespoons raw almonds
- ½ cup ice cubes

Instructions:

1. Combine all ingredients in a blender.
2. Blend on high speed for 30 to 60 seconds until smooth.
3. Pour into glasses and serve immediately.

Vanilla Coconut Smoothie

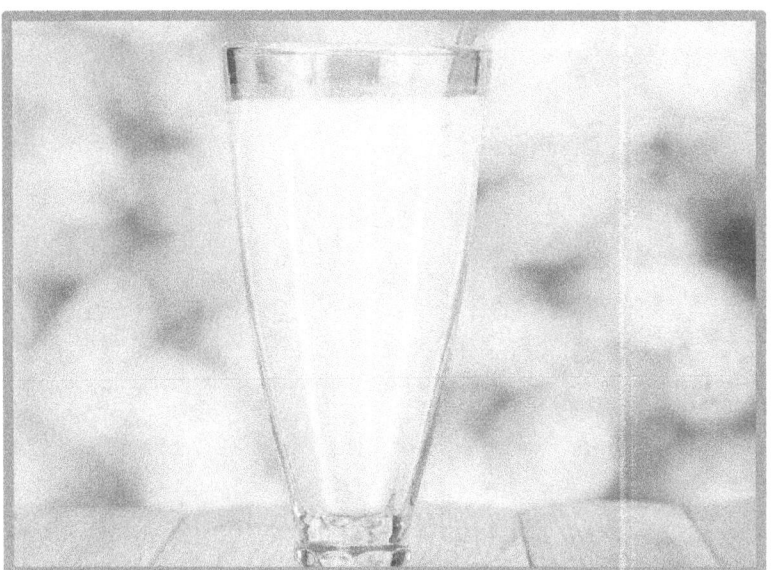

Servings: 2

Ingredients:

- 1 frozen green-tipped banana, sliced
- 1 cup unsweetened coconut milk
- ¼ cup unsweetened shredded coconut
- ½ cup ice cubes
- ¼ teaspoon vanilla extract

Instructions:

1. Combine all ingredients in a blender.
2. Blend on high speed for 30 to 60 seconds until smooth.
3. Pour into glasses and serve immediately.

3-Ingredient Banana Pancakes

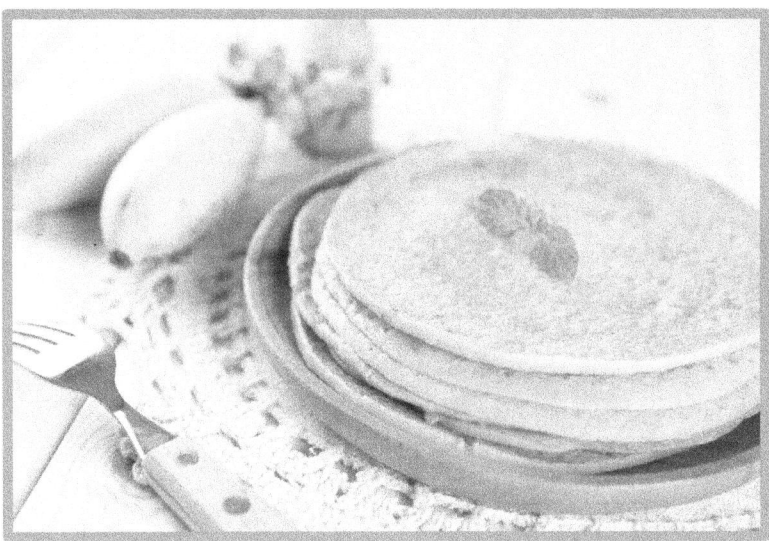

Servings: 2

Ingredients:

- 3 large green-tipped bananas, peeled and chopped
- 4 large eggs, lightly beaten
- ¼ teaspoon baking powder

Instructions:

1. Combine all of the ingredients in a food processor and blend until smooth.
2. Heat a medium skillet over medium-high heat and grease with cooking spray.
3. Spoon the batter into the skillet in heaping tablespoons.
4. Cook the pancakes for 1 to 2 minutes until the undersides are brown.
5. Carefully flip the pancakes and cook for 1 to 2 minutes more until lightly browned.
6. Transfer the pancakes to a plate to keep warm and repeat with the remaining batter.
7. Serve hot with extra banana slices, if desired.

Spiced Pumpkin Pancakes

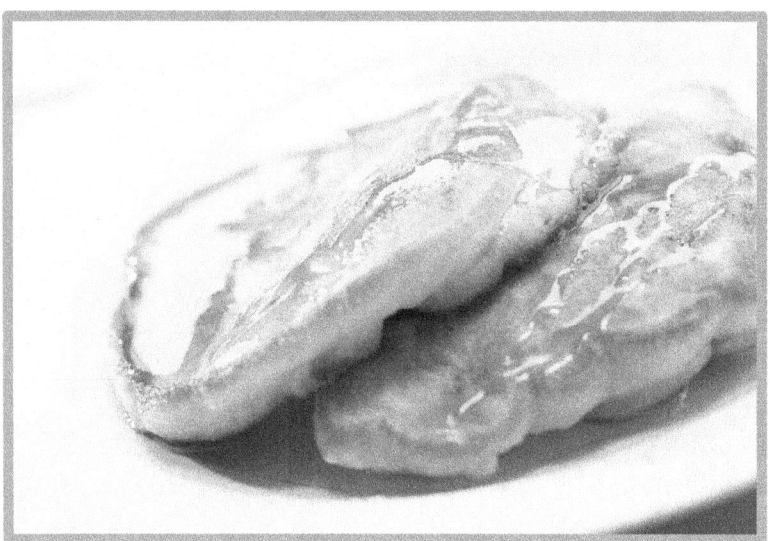

Servings: 2

Ingredients:

- 2/3 cup almond flour
- ½ cup pumpkin puree
- 2 large eggs, lightly beaten
- ¾ teaspoon ground cinnamon
- ¼ teaspoon ground nutmeg
- ¼ teaspoon baking soda
- ¼ teaspoon vanilla extract
- Pinch salt

Instructions:

1. Whisk together the pumpkin, eggs and vanilla extract in a small mixing bowl.
2. In a separate bowl, combine the almond flour, cinnamon, nutmeg, baking soda and salt.
3. Add the wet ingredients to the dry and whisk until smooth and well combined.
4. Grease a medium skillet and heat it over medium-high heat.
5. Spoon the batter into the skillet in heaping tablespoons.
6. Cook the pancakes for 1 to 2 minutes until lightly browned on the undersides then flip and cook until brown on the other side.
7. Transfer the pancakes to a plate and repeat with the remaining batter.

Easy Almond Flour Muffins

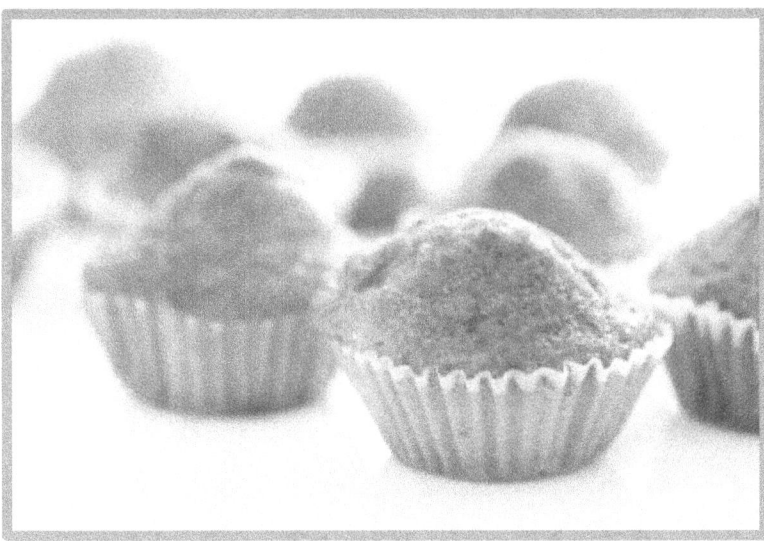

Servings: makes 12 muffins

Ingredients:

- 3 cups almond flour
- 6 large eggs, lightly beaten
- 2 teaspoons apple cider vinegar
- 1 teaspoon baking soda
- Pinch salt

Instructions:

1. Preheat the oven to 350°F and line a regular muffin pan with paper liners.
2. Combine the almond flour, baking soda and salt in a mixing bowl.
3. In a separate bowl, beat together the eggs and apple cider vinegar until smooth.
4. Add the dry ingredients to the wet and blend until well combined.
5. If desired, fold in some chopped nuts or banana.
6. Spoon the batter into the prepared pan, filling the cups about 2/3 full.
7. Bake for 15 minutes until the muffins are lightly browned around the edges.
8. Cool the muffins for 20 minutes or so before serving.

Tomato Basil Omelet

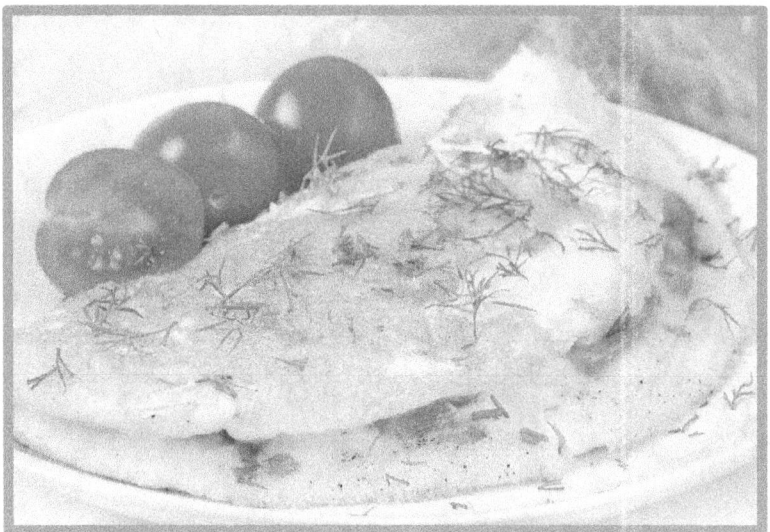

Servings: 1

Ingredients:

- 2 large eggs
- ½ teaspoon salt
- ¼ teaspoon fresh black pepper
- 2 teaspoons olive oil
- 1 medium ripe tomato, chopped
- 4 fresh basil leaves, chopped
- Fresh chopped dill

Instructions:

1. Whisk together the eggs, salt and pepper in a small bowl and set aside.
2. Heat 1 teaspoon olive oil in a medium skillet over medium-high heat.
3. Add the tomato and basil and cook for 2 minutes, stirring often.
4. Spoon the tomato and basil into a bowl.
5. Heat the remaining teaspoon of olive oil in the skillet and pour in the egg mixture.
6. Cook for 2 minutes, scraping down the sides of the skillet as needed to spread the uncooked egg.
7. When the egg is almost set, spoon the tomato basil mixture over half the omelet.
8. Fold the empty half of the omelet over the fillings and cook for 1 minute more.
9. Slide the omelet onto a plate and garnish with fresh dill to serve.

Mushroom Scallion Omelet

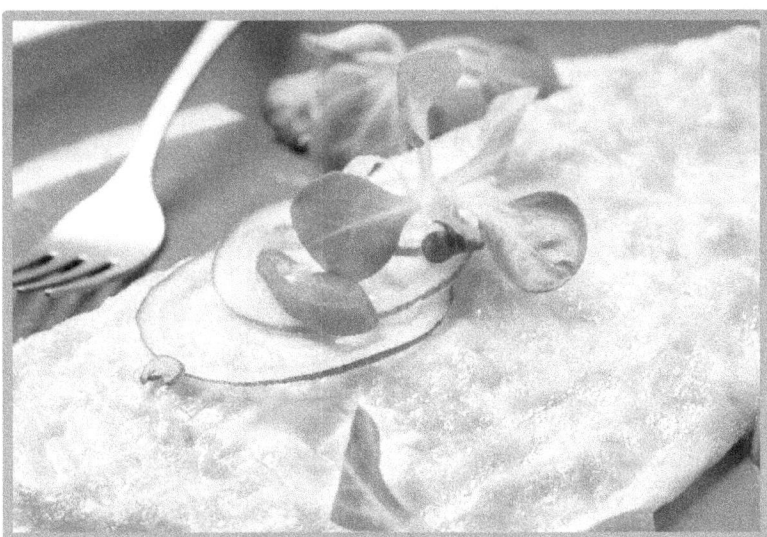

Servings: 1

Ingredients:

- 2 large eggs
- ½ teaspoon salt
- ¼ teaspoon fresh black pepper
- 2 teaspoons olive oil
- 1 cup diced mushrooms
- 2 scallions, sliced thin

Instructions:

1. Whisk together the eggs, salt and pepper in a small bowl and set aside.
2. Heat 1 teaspoon olive oil in a medium skillet over medium-high heat.
3. Add the mushrooms and scallions and cook for 3 minutes, stirring often.
4. Spoon the mushroom and scallions into a bowl.
5. Heat the remaining teaspoon of olive oil in the skillet and pour in the egg mixture.
6. Cook for 2 minutes, scraping down the sides of the skillet as needed to spread the uncooked egg.
7. When the egg is almost set, spoon the mushroom scallion mixture over half the omelet.
8. Fold the empty half of the omelet over the fillings and cook for 1 minute more.
9. Slide the omelet onto a plate to serve.

Lunch Recipes

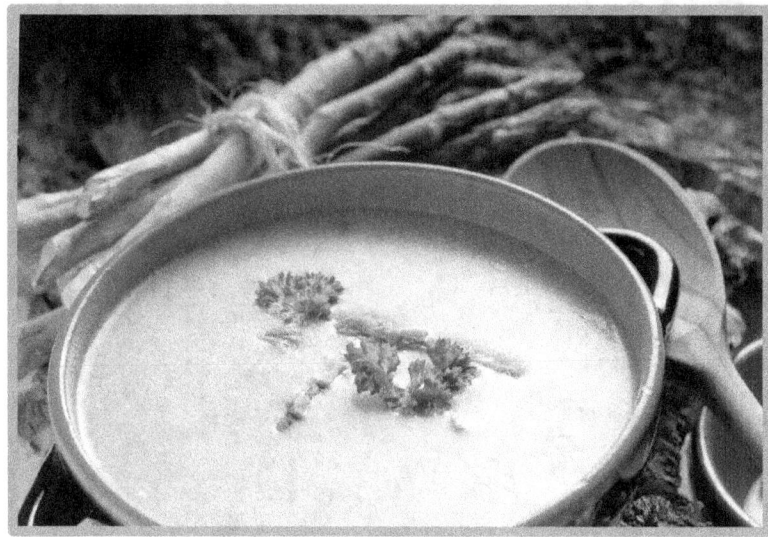

The recipes included in this section are full of flavor but easy to prepare – the perfect option for lunch on your sugar detox. Here you will find everything from cream of cauliflower soup to a fresh spring salad with homemade balsamic dressing.

Recipes Included in this Section:

Cream of Cauliflower Soup

Chilled Avocado Soup

Creamy Curried Carrot Soup

Hearty Chicken Vegetable Soup

Avocado Kale Salad with Almonds

Warm Quinoa Vegetable Salad

Spring Salad with Balsamic Dressing

Chilled Three-Bean Salad

Cream of Cauliflower Soup

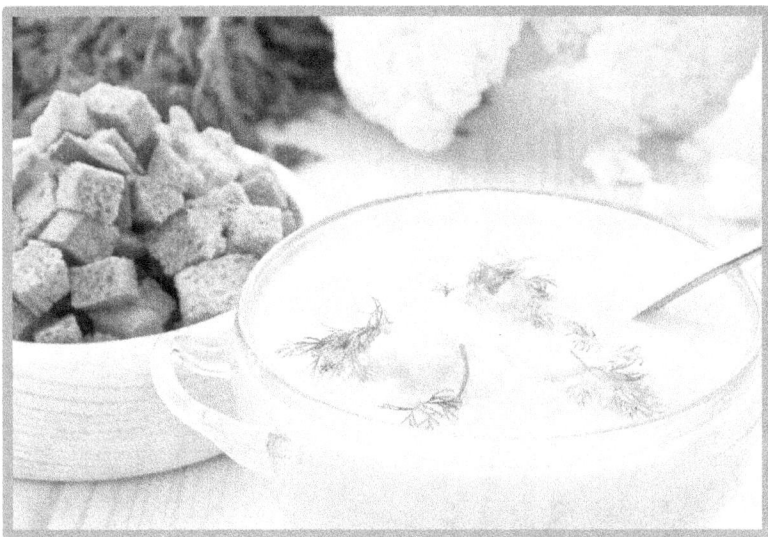

Servings: 4 to 6

Ingredients:

- 2 lbs. cauliflower, chopped
- 2 tablespoons olive oil
- 1 large yellow onion, chopped
- 1 teaspoon minced garlic
- 4 cups chicken broth
- Salt and pepper to taste
- 1 cup canned coconut milk
- Fresh dill to serve

Instructions:

1. Heat the oil in a stock pot over medium heat.
2. Add the onions and garlic and cook until the onions are tender, about 8 to 10 minutes.
3. Stir in the cauliflower and chicken broth – top off with water if the cauliflower isn't covered.
4. Bring the soup to a boil then simmer, covered, for 20 minutes until the cauliflower is tender.
5. Season with salt and pepper to taste then remove from heat and puree the soup using an immersion blender.
6. Whisk in the coconut milk then serve hot, garnished with fresh dill.

Chilled Avocado Soup

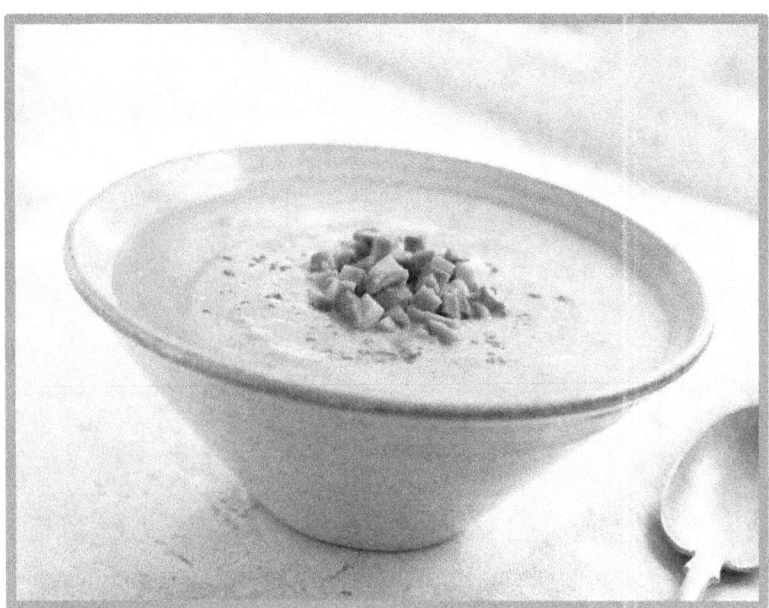

Servings: 4

Ingredients:

- 1 small seedless cucumber, peeled and diced
- 1 ripe avocado, pitted and chopped
- 1 shallot, diced
- 2 tablespoons canned coconut milk
- 2 tablespoons fresh chopped mint
- 1 tablespoon fresh lime juice
- Salt and pepper to taste

Instructions:

1. Combine all of the ingredients in a food processor and blend until smooth.
2. Cover and chill for at least 1 hour before serving.

Creamy Curried Carrot Soup

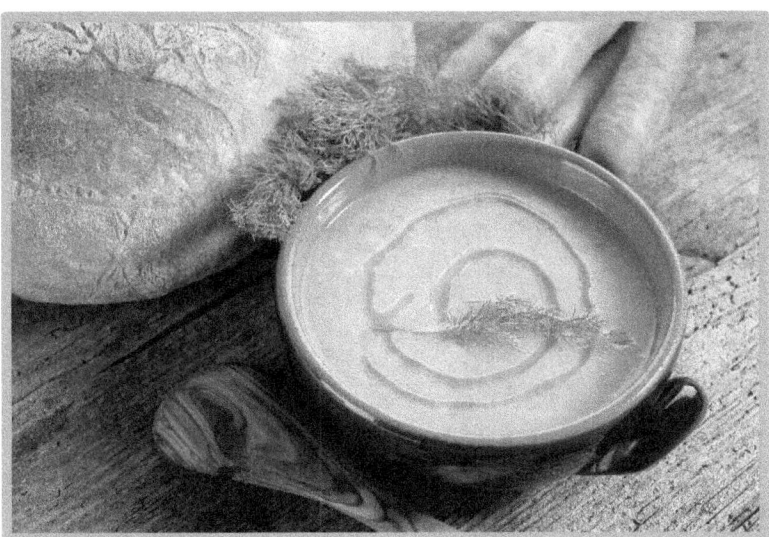

Servings: 4 to 6

Ingredients:

- 2 tablespoons olive oil
- 2 teaspoons curry powder
- 1 teaspoon minced garlic
- 8 large carrots, peeled and chopped
- 1 large yellow onion, chopped
- 2 large stalks celery, chopped
- 5 cups vegetable or chicken broth
- Salt and pepper to taste

Instructions:

1. Heat the olive oil in a stockpot over medium heat.
2. Add the curry powder and garlic and cook for 1 minute, stirring.
3. Stir in the carrots, onion, celery and broth then bring to a boil.
4. Reduce heat and simmer for 20 minutes until the carrots are very tender.
5. Remove from heat and puree using an immersion blender.
6. Season the soup with salt and pepper to serve.

Hearty Chicken Vegetable Soup

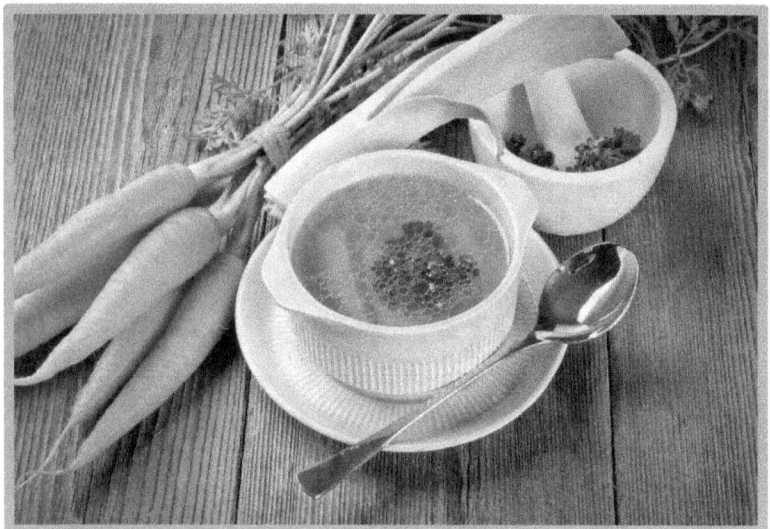

Servings: 4 to 6

Ingredients:

- 2 tablespoons olive oil
- 1 tablespoon minced garlic
- 1 large yellow onion, chopped
- 2 large carrots, peeled and sliced
- 2 large stalks celery, sliced
- 2 cups broccoli florets
- 2 boneless skinless chicken breasts, chopped
- 8 cups chicken broth
- 2 tablespoons fresh chopped parsley
- 1 teaspoon dried oregano
- 1 teaspoon fresh chopped tarragon
- Salt and pepper to taste

Instructions:

1. Heat the oil in a stockpot over medium heat.
2. Add the garlic and cook for 1 minute.
3. Stir in the onion, carrots, celery and broccoli and cook for 10 minutes, stirring occasionally, until the onions are tender.
4. Add the chicken broth, parsley, oregano and tarragon then bring to a boil.
5. Reduce heat and simmer for 15 minutes until the chicken is cooked through.

6. Season with salt and pepper to taste.

Avocado Kale Salad with Almonds

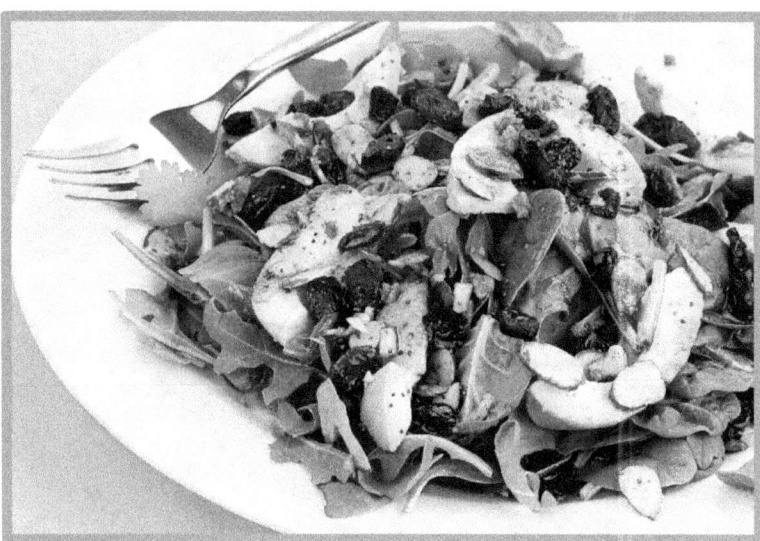

Servings: 2

Ingredients:

- 4 cups fresh chopped kale
- ½ ripe avocado, pitted and sliced thin
- 3 tablespoons sliced almonds
- 2 tablespoons olive oil
- 1 tablespoon red wine vinegar
- 1 tablespoon balsamic vinegar
- Pinch dry mustard powder
- Salt and pepper to taste

Instructions:

1. Divide the kale between two plates and top with sliced avocado and almonds.
2. Whisk together the remaining ingredients in a small bowl then drizzle over the salads to serve.

Warm Quinoa Vegetable Salad

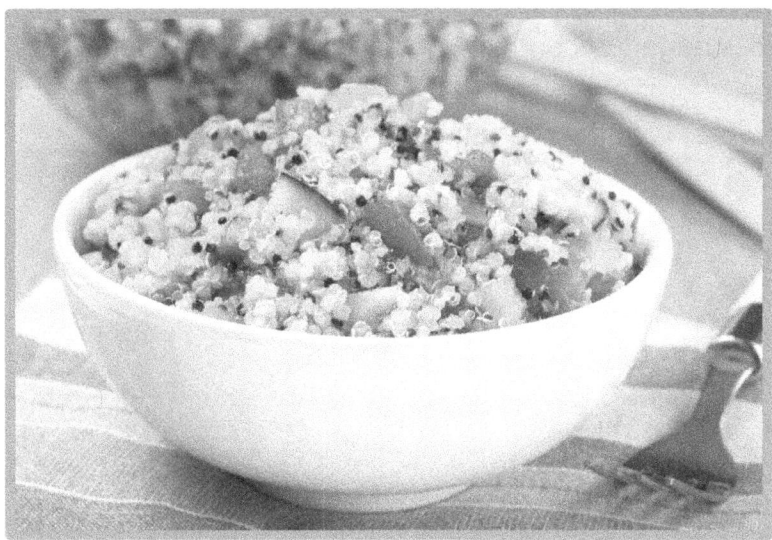

Servings: 6 to 8

Ingredients:

- 1 tablespoon coconut oil
- 1 small yellow onion, chopped
- 1 small zucchini, diced
- ½ red bell pepper, cored and chopped
- ½ yellow bell pepper, cored and chopped
- 1 ¼ cups dry quinoa
- Water as needed
- 3 tablespoons olive oil
- 3 tablespoons red wine vinegar
- 1 tablespoon coconut aminos
- ¼ cup sliced scallions
- ¼ cup fresh chopped cilantro

Instructions:

1. Heat the oil in a medium skillet over medium-high heat.
2. Add the onion, zucchini, red pepper and yellow pepper and cook for 4 to 5 minutes until just tender.
3. Set the vegetables aside to cool slightly.
4. Place the quinoa in a medium saucepan and cover it with about 2 inches of water.

5. Bring the water to a boil then reduce to medium-low and simmer, uncovered, for 15 minutes until the quinoa has popped.
6. Set the quinoa aside to cool.
7. Whisk together the olive oil, vinegar, coconut aminos, cilantro and scallions in a small bowl.
8. Toss the quinoa and vegetables with the dressing to serve.

Spring Salad with Balsamic Dressing

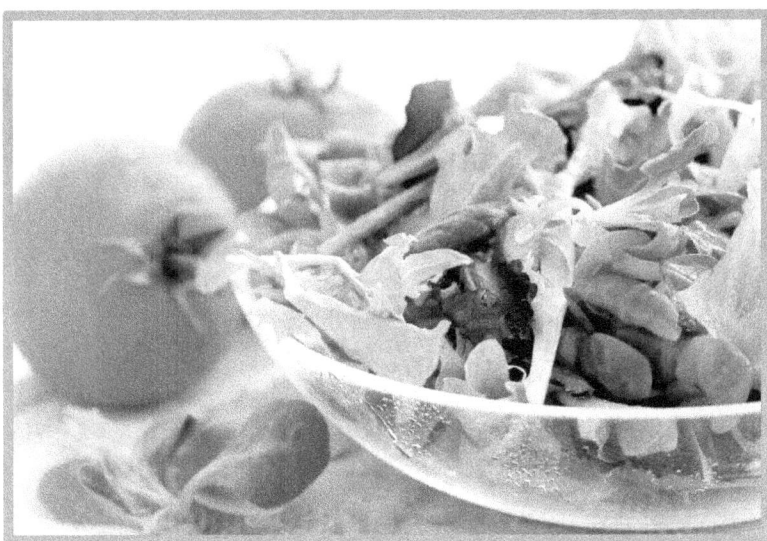

Servings: 2

Ingredients:

- 4 cups fresh spring greens
- 1 small ripe tomato, chopped
- ¼ cup thinly sliced red onion
- 2 tablespoons extra-virgin olive oil
- 2 tablespoons balsamic vinegar
- 1 tablespoon minced yellow onion
- Pinch dry mustard powder
- Salt and pepper to taste

Instructions:

1. Combine the spring greens, onion and tomato in a salad bowl.
2. Whisk together the remaining ingredients in small bowl then toss with the salad to serve.

Chilled Three-Bean Salad

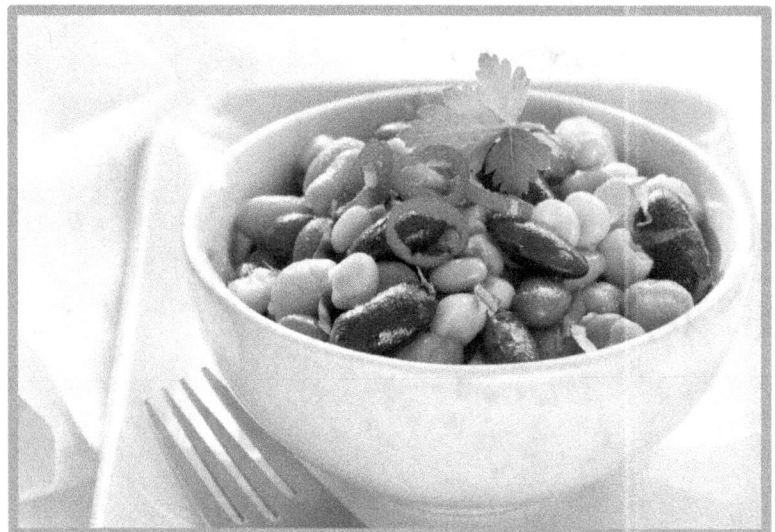

Servings: 4 to 6

Ingredients:

- 1 (15 ounce) can white cannellini beans, rinsed and drained
- 1 (15 ounce) can red kidney beans, rinsed and drained
- 1 (15 ounce) can chickpeas, rinsed and drained
- ½ small red onion, diced
- 1 cup fresh chopped parsley
- 2 tablespoons fresh chopped cilantro
- 1/3 cup apple cider vinegar
- ¼ cup extra-virgin olive oil
- Salt and pepper to taste

Instructions:

1. Combine the beans, red onion, parsley and cilantro in a large mixing bowl and stir well.
2. Toss with the vinegar, olive oil, salt and pepper.
3. Chill until ready to serve.

Dinner Recipes

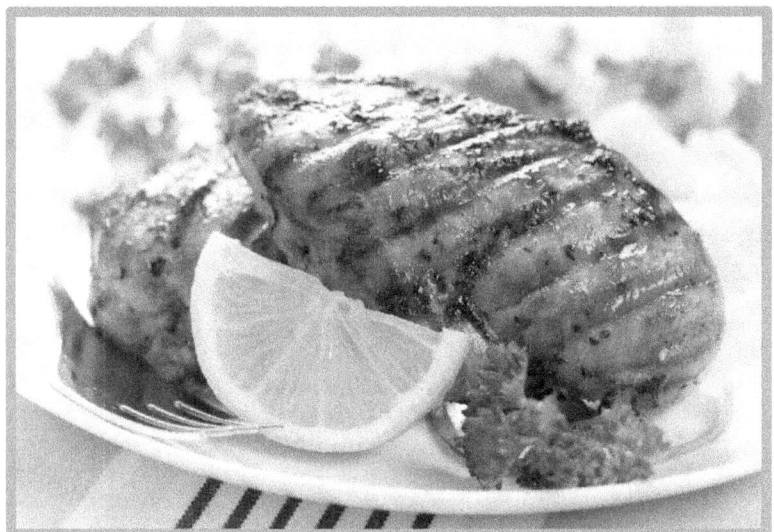

While you are engaging in the sugar detox, you may be surprised to find just how many delicious and flavorful dishes can be made without any sugar at all. The recipes in this section are guaranteed to fill your stomach and satisfy your hunger, all without a single gram of sugar.

<u>Recipes Included in this Section:</u>

Rosemary Roasted Chicken Legs

Coconut-Crusted Baked Halibut

Balsamic-Glazed Pork Chops

Bacon-Wrapped Scallops

Slow-Cooker Beef Stew

Chicken and Vegetable Curry

Baked Haddock with Fresh Salsa

Spicy Seafood Soup

Rosemary Roasted Chicken Legs

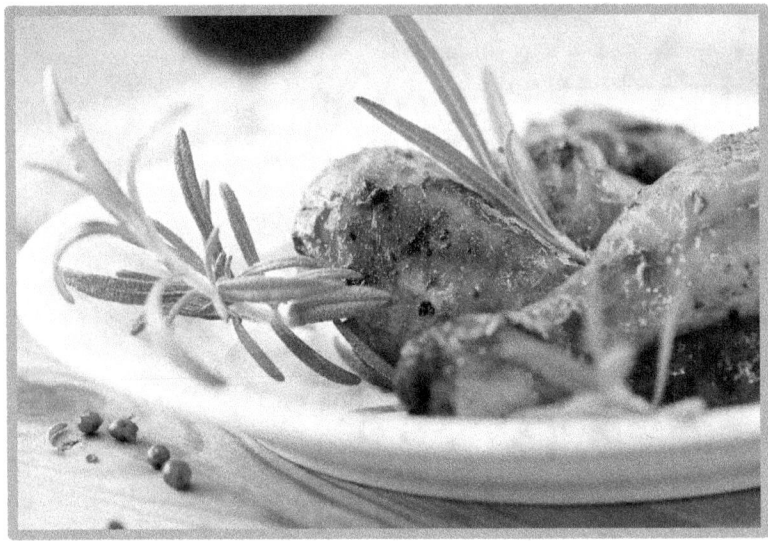

Servings: 4

Ingredients:

- 2 lbs. bone-in chicken thighs and drumsticks
- 1 tablespoon coconut oil
- Salt and pepper to taste
- ¼ cup chicken broth
- 2 tablespoons dried rosemary

Instructions:

1. Heat the coconut oil in a large skillet over medium-high heat.
2. Season the chicken with salt and pepper to taste and add to the skillet.
3. Cook the chicken for 2 minutes on each side until lightly browned then transfer to a glass baking dish.
4. Drizzle with chicken broth and sprinkle with rosemary.
5. Roast for 30 minutes then turn the chicken and roast for another 20 to 30 minutes until the juices run clear.

Coconut-Crusted Baked Halibut

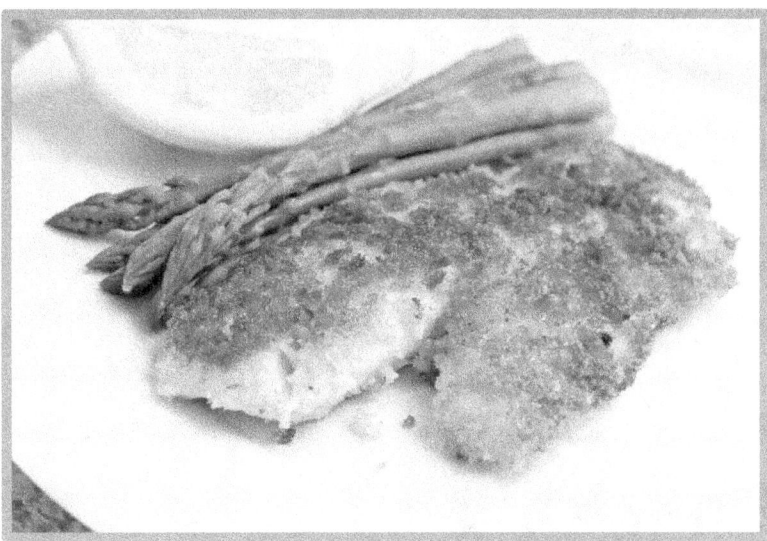

Servings: 4

Ingredients:

- 4 (6-ounce) boneless halibut fillets
- ¼ cup coconut flour
- ¼ cup unsweetened shredded coconut
- Salt and pepper to taste
- 1 large egg, lightly beaten
- Lemon wedges

Instructions:

1. Preheat the oven to 350°F.
2. Combine the coconut flour, coconut, salt and pepper in a small bowl.
3. Dip the fillets in the beaten egg then coat with the coconut flour mixture.
4. Place the fillets on a parchment-lined baking sheet and bake for 12 to 15 minutes until the flesh flakes easily with a fork.
5. Serve the fish hot with lemon wedges.

Balsamic-Glazed Pork Chops

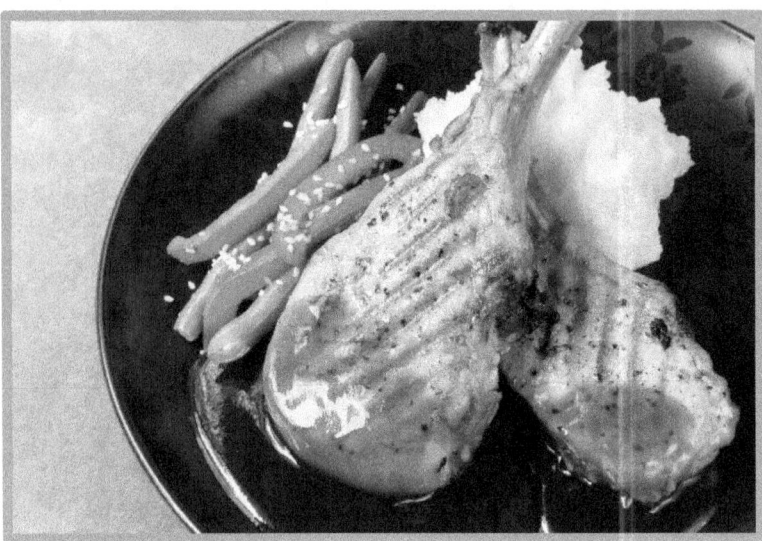

Servings: 4

Ingredients:

- 4 (6-ounce) bone-in pork chops
- Salt and pepper to taste
- 3 tablespoons balsamic vinegar
- 1 tablespoon olive oil

Instructions:

1. Preheat the broiler in your oven to high heat.
2. Whisk together the balsamic vinegar and olive oil in a small bowl.
3. Season the chops with salt and pepper to taste then brush with the balsamic mixture.
4. Broil the chops for 7 to 8 minutes until browned.
5. Brush the chops with more balsamic mixture and flip them.
6. Cook for another 7 to 8 minutes until cooked to the desired level.

Bacon-Wrapped Scallops

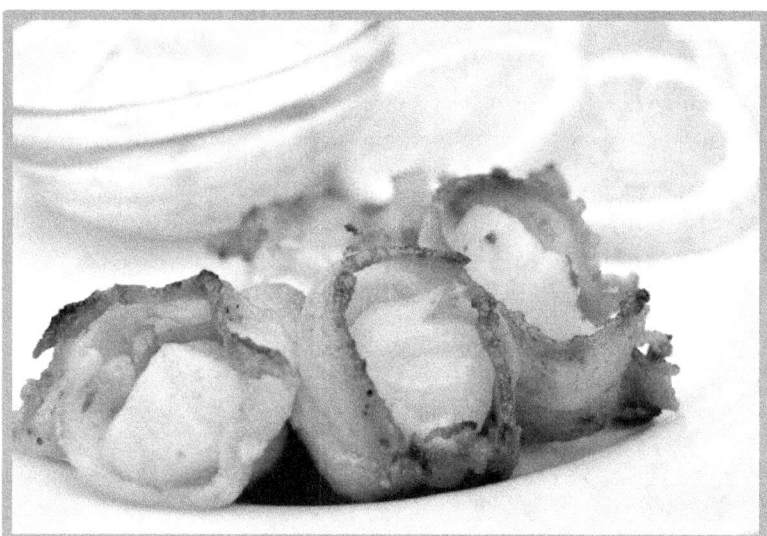

Servings: 4

Ingredients:

- 1 ½ lbs. raw sea scallops
- 1 lbs. uncooked bacon
- 1 teaspoon chili powder
- Salt and pepper to taste

Instructions:

1. Preheat the broiler in your oven to high heat.
2. Rinse the scallops well then pat them dry.
3. Wrap each scallop in a slice of bacon and secure it in place with a wooden toothpick.
4. Season the scallops with chili powder, salt and pepper then place them under the broiler.
5. Broil for 3 to 5 minutes on each side until the bacon is crisp.

Slow-Cooker Beef Stew

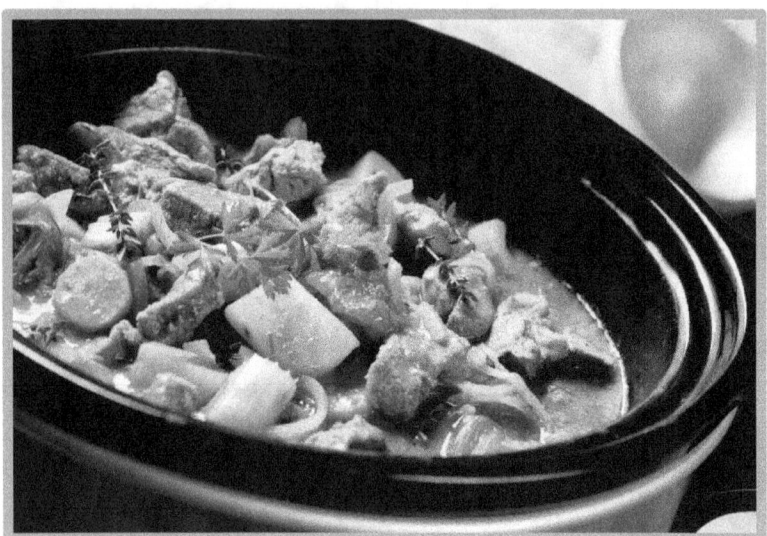

Servings: 4 to 6

Ingredients:

- 2 lbs. beef stew meat
- 1 tablespoon coconut oil
- Salt and pepper to taste
- 1 large onion, quartered
- 2 stalks celery, sliced
- 2 cups baby carrots
- 1 medium parsnip, peeled and chopped
- 1 tablespoon dried parsley
- 1 teaspoon dried oregano
- 8 cups beef broth or stock
- ¼ cup almond flour
- ¼ cup water

Instructions:

1. Heat the coconut oil in a large skillet over medium-high heat.
2. Add the beef and cook until browned, stirring as needed.
3. Transfer the beef to the slow cooker and stir in the onion, celery, carrots, parsnip, parsley and oregano.
4. Stir in the beef broth then cover and cook on low heat for 10 hours or on high heat for 6 to 7 hours.

5. Whisk together the water and almond flour then stir into the slow cooker and cook for another 30 minutes or so until thickened.

Chicken and Vegetable Curry

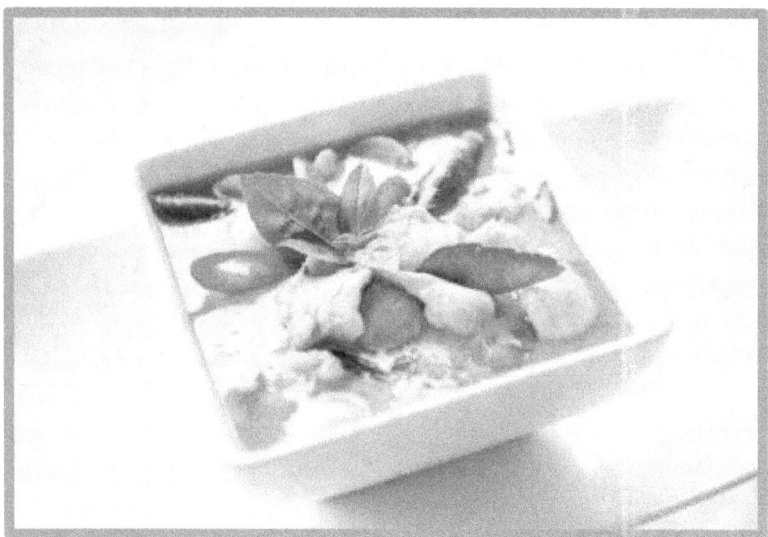

Servings: 4

Ingredients:

- 2 tablespoons olive oil
- 3 tablespoons red curry paste
- 1 large yellow onion, sliced
- 2 boneless skinless chicken breasts, cut into 1-inch chunks
- 1 cup broccoli florets
- 1 cup sliced carrots
- ½ medium red pepper, cored and chopped
- 1 tablespoon fresh lime zest
- 1 ¼ cups canned coconut milk
- ¼ cup chicken broth
- 1 (14-ounce) can diced tomatoes

Instructions:

1. Heat the olive oil in a large skillet over medium heat.
2. Add the onions and curry paste and stir well – cook for 5 to 6 minutes until the onions are translucent.
3. Add the chicken and season with salt and pepper to taste.
4. Cook for 2 to 3 minutes on each side until the chicken is lightly browned.
5. Stir in the broccoli, carrots and red pepper and lime zest.

6. Whisk in the coconut milk, chicken broth and tomatoes then bring the mixture to a gentle simmer.
7. Simmer for 20 minutes until the sauce is thickened. Serve hot.

Baked Haddock with Fresh Salsa

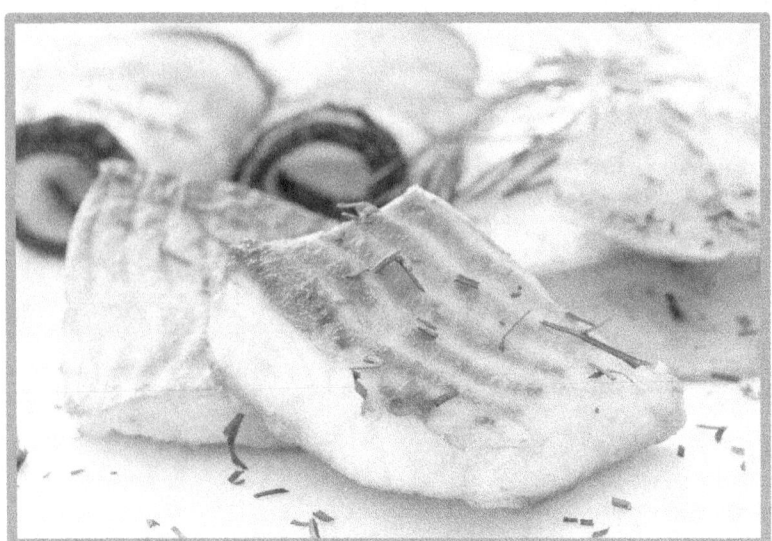

Servings: 4

Ingredients:

- 4 (6-ounce) boneless haddock fillets
- 1 tablespoon olive oil
- Salt and pepper to taste
- 2 medium ripe tomatoes, diced
- ½ medium green pepper, cored and diced
- ½ jalapeno pepper, seeded minced
- ¼ cup fresh chopped cilantro
- 1 teaspoon salt
- ½ teaspoon ground cumin

Instructions:

1. Preheat the oven to 350°F and line a baking sheet with parchment.
2. Brush the fillets with olive oil and season with salt and pepper to taste.
3. Bake the fillets for 12 to 15 minutes until the flesh flakes easily with a fork.
4. Meanwhile, combine the remaining ingredients in a bowl and toss to combine.
5. Serve the fish hot with fresh salsa over top.

Spicy Seafood Soup

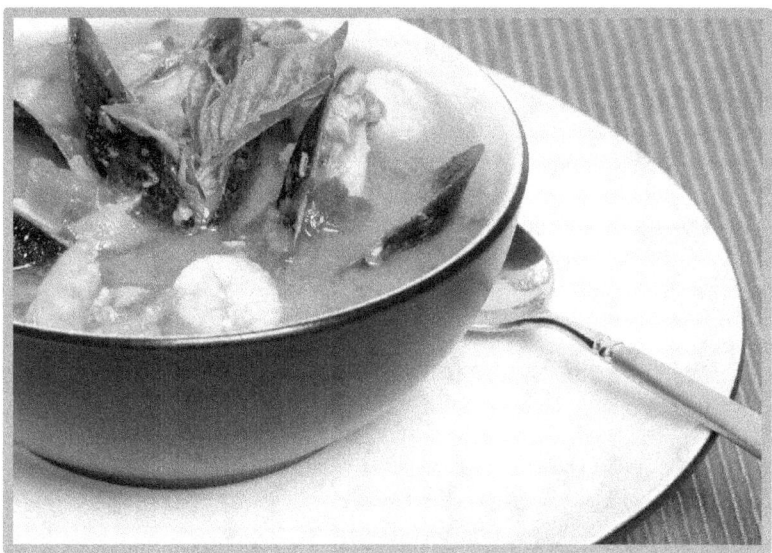

Servings: 4

Ingredients:

- 8 cups chicken broth
- 2 cups sliced mushrooms
- ½ cup chopped kale
- 2 (4 to 6-ounce) tilapia fillets, cut into 1-inch chunks
- 12 raw shrimp, peeled and deveined
- 12 raw mussels, rinsed well
- 1 cup canned coconut milk
- Salt to taste

Instructions:

1. Bring the chicken broth to a boil in a stockpot over high heat.
2. Stir in the mushrooms and kale then bring to a boil again.
3. Add the shrimp, fish and mussels and let the soup come to a boil.
4. Boil the soup for 3 to 4 minutes until the shrimp turn pink then stir in the coconut milk and salt to taste.
5. Cook the soup until just heated through then serve hot.

Snack Recipes

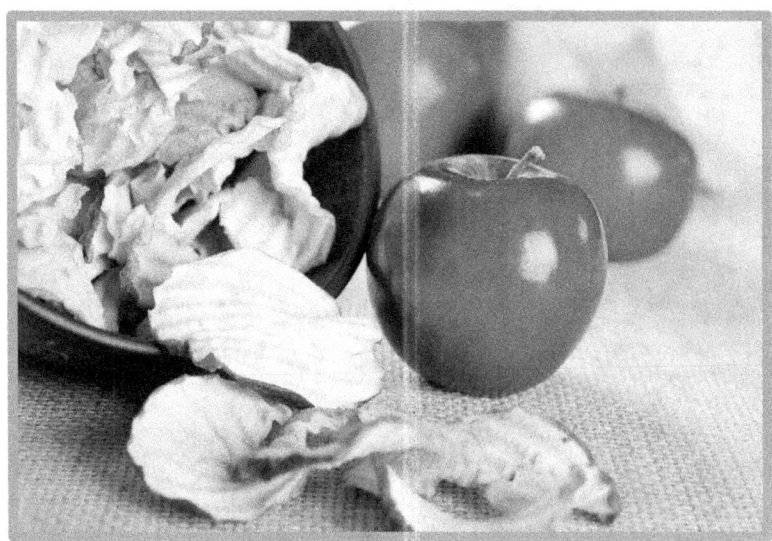

Just because you are engaging in a sugar detox doesn't mean that you have to give up tasty snacks. In this section you will find recipes for a variety of delicious treats from baked banana chips to chocolate mousse.

Recipes Included in this Section:

Crispy Kale Chips

Cinnamon Baked Banana Chips

Sweet and Salty Trail Mix

Spicy Mixed Nuts

Avocado Chocolate Mousse

Baked Apples with Walnuts

Mini Banana Nut Muffins

Roasted Cauliflower Bites

Crispy Kale Chips

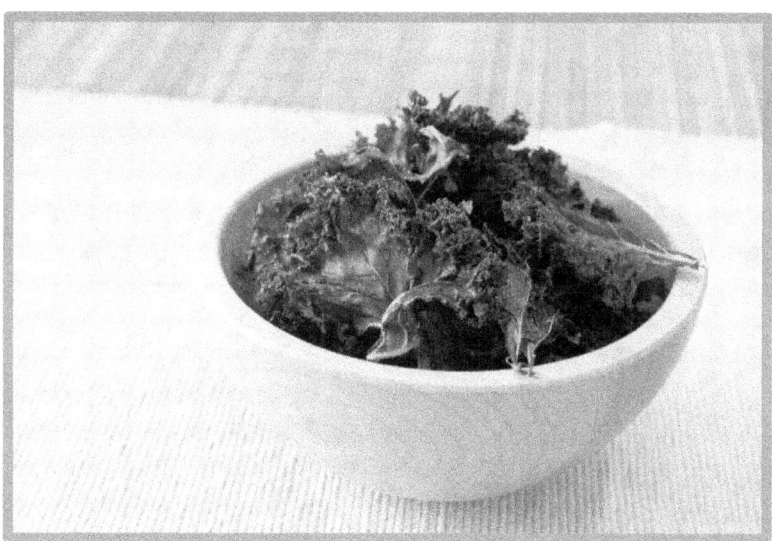

Servings: 3

Ingredients:

- 2 large bunches fresh kale
- 2 tablespoons olive oil
- Salt and pepper to taste

Instructions:

1. Preheat the oven to 350°F.
2. Tear the kale into 2-inch chunks by hand and toss with olive oil.
3. Spread the kale on parchment-lined baking sheets and season with salt and pepper to taste.
4. Bake for 12 to 15 minutes until dry and crisp.

Cinnamon Baked Banana Chips

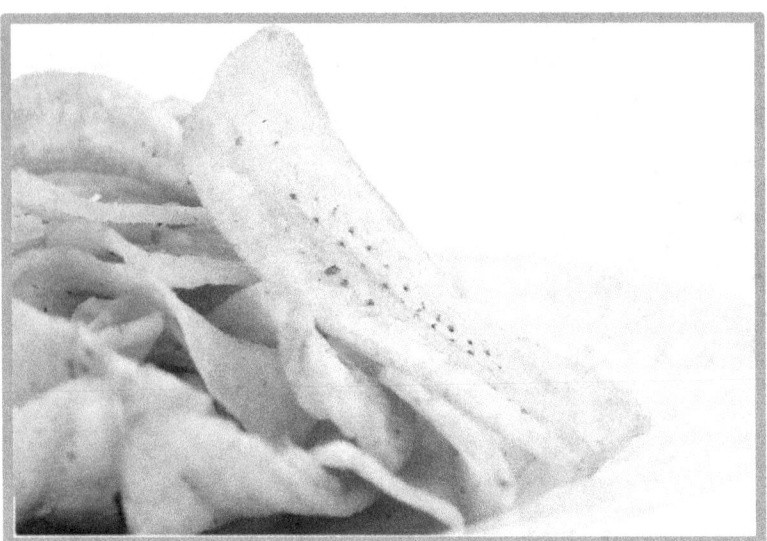

Servings: 2

Ingredients:

- 3 large green-tipped bananas, peeled and sliced
- 1 tablespoon fresh lemon juice
- Pinch ground cinnamon

Instructions:

1. Preheat the oven to 250°F.
2. Toss the banana slices with lemon juice and cinnamon.
3. Spread the slices on a parchment-lined baking sheet and bake for 1 ½ hours, flipping halfway through.
4. Turn off the oven and let the slices sit until crisp.

Sweet and Salty Trail Mix

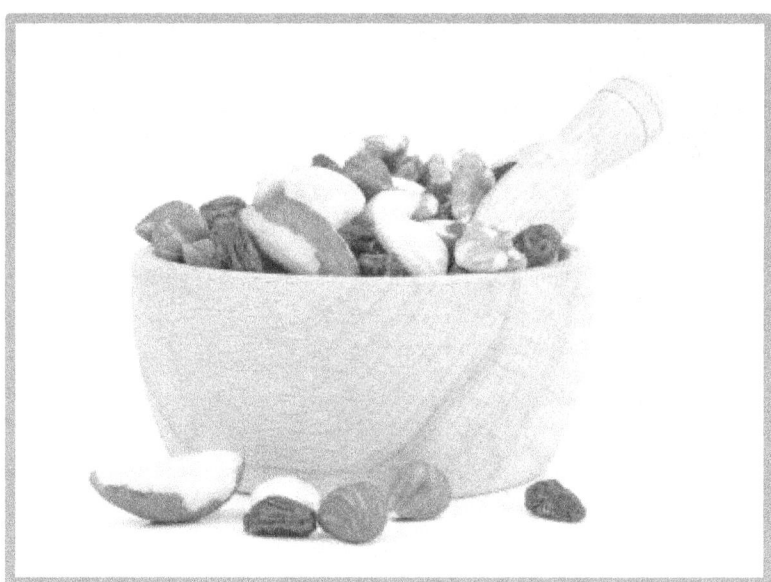

Servings: 4

Ingredients:

- 1 cup hulled sunflower seeds
- 1 cup hulled pumpkin seeds
- ½ cup raw almonds
- ½ cup raw pecans
- ½ cup unsweetened flaked coconut
- ½ cup chopped banana chips
- 1 teaspoon coarse salt
- Pinch chili powder

Instructions:

1. Combine the seeds, nuts, coconut and banana chips in a bowl and toss to combine.
2. Toss with the salt and chili powder to coat and serve.

Spicy Mixed Nuts

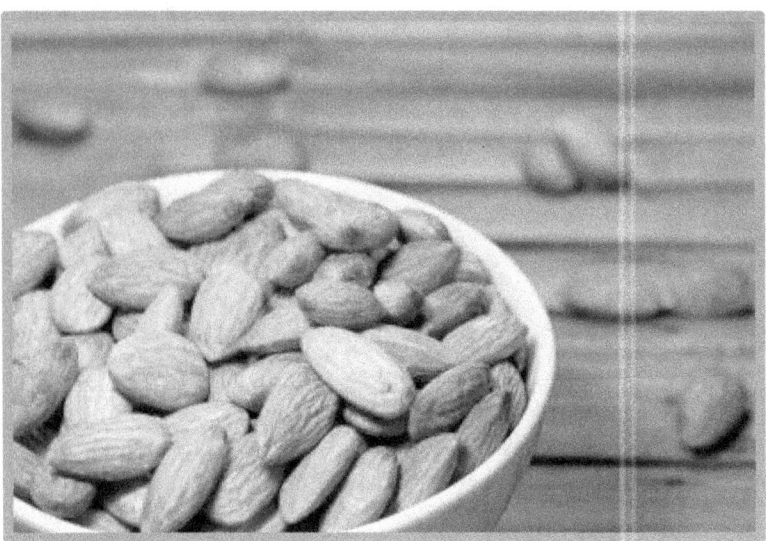

Servings: 4

Ingredients:

- 1 cup raw almonds
- ½ cup raw pecans (whole)
- ½ cup raw walnuts (halves)
- 1 teaspoon chili powder
- 1 teaspoon salt
- ½ teaspoon fresh black pepper
- Pinch cayenne pepper
- 1 tablespoon olive oil

Instructions:

1. Combine the nuts in a large skillet over medium heat.
2. Let the nuts cook for 4 to 5 minutes, stirring often, until they are lightly toasted.
3. Combine the chili powder, salt, pepper and cayenne in a small bowl.
4. Toss the hot nuts with the olive oil and the spice mixture to coat.
5. Cool the nuts before serving.

Avocado Chocolate Mousse

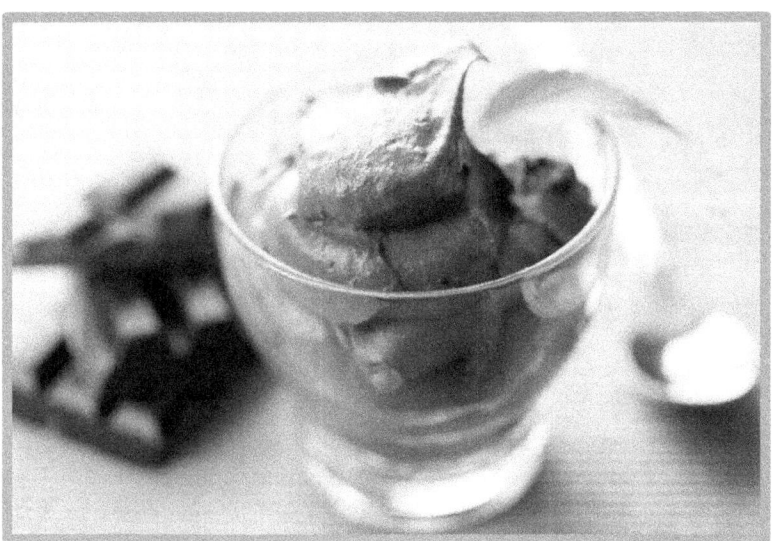

Servings: 4

Ingredients:

- 2 ripe avocados, pitted and chopped
- ¼ cup unsweetened cocoa powder
- ½ teaspoon vanilla extract

Instructions:

1. Combine all of the ingredients in a food processor and blend until smooth.
2. Spoon into dessert cups and chill until ready to serve.

Baked Apples with Walnuts

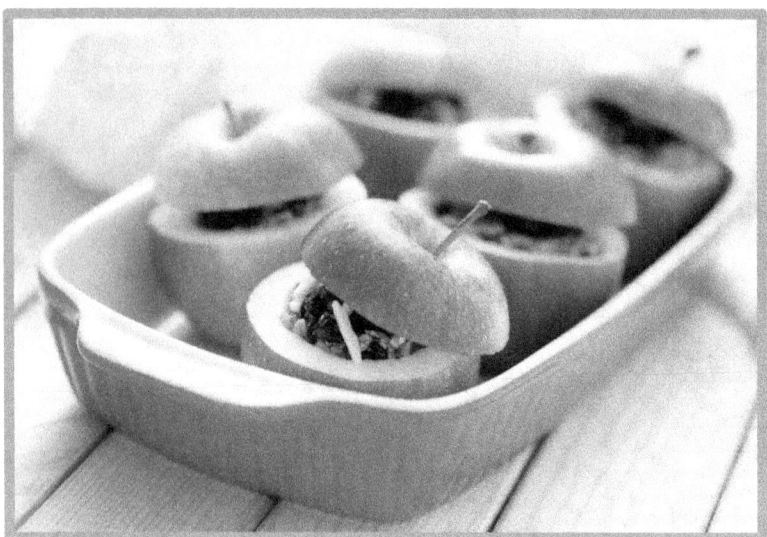

Servings: 4

Ingredients:

- 4 ripe Granny Smith apples
- ¼ cup almond flour
- ¼ cup chopped walnuts
- 2 tablespoon coconut oil
- 1 teaspoon ground cinnamon
- Pinch ground nutmeg

Instructions:

1. Preheat the oven to 350°F.
2. Cut the tops off the apples with a sharp knife and carefully remove the core.
3. Combine the almond flour, walnuts, coconut oil, cinnamon and nutmeg in a small bowl.
4. Spoon the filling into the cored apples then place them in a glass baking dish.
5. Bake for 30 minutes until the apples are hot and tender.

Mini Banana Nut Muffins

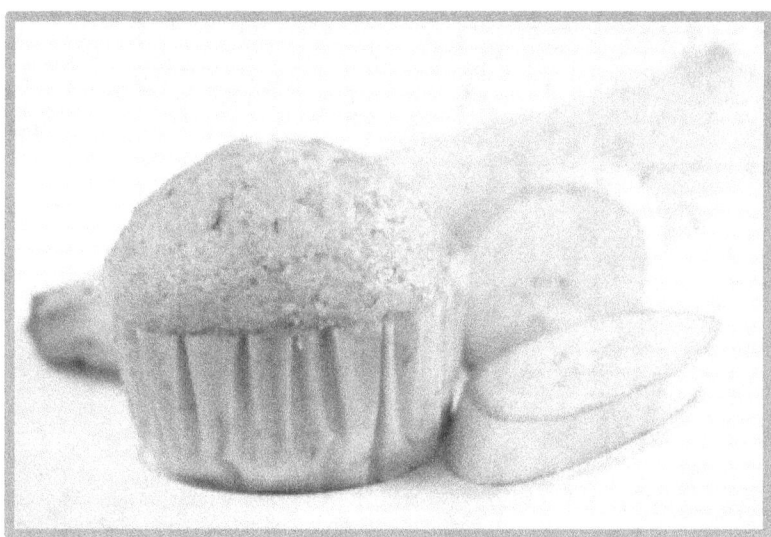

Servings: 24

Ingredients:

- 4 medium green-tipped bananas, peeled and chopped
- ½ cup coconut flour, sifted
- 4 large eggs, lightly beaten
- ½ cup natural almond butter
- 2 tablespoons melted coconut oil
- 2 teaspoons ground cinnamon
- 1 teaspoon baking powder
- ¾ teaspoons baking soda
- Pinch salt
- ½ cup finely chopped walnuts

Instructions:

1. Preheat the oven to 350°F and line a 24-cup mini muffin pan with paper liners.
2. Mash the bananas in a large mixing bowl and whisk in the eggs, almond butter and coconut oil.
3. In a separate bowl, combine the coconut flour, cinnamon, baking powder, baking soda and salt.
4. Blend the dry ingredients into the wet until smooth and well combined.
5. Fold in the walnuts then drop the batter into the prepared pan.
6. Bake for 18 to 22 minutes until a knife inserted in the center comes out clean.

Roasted Cauliflower Bites

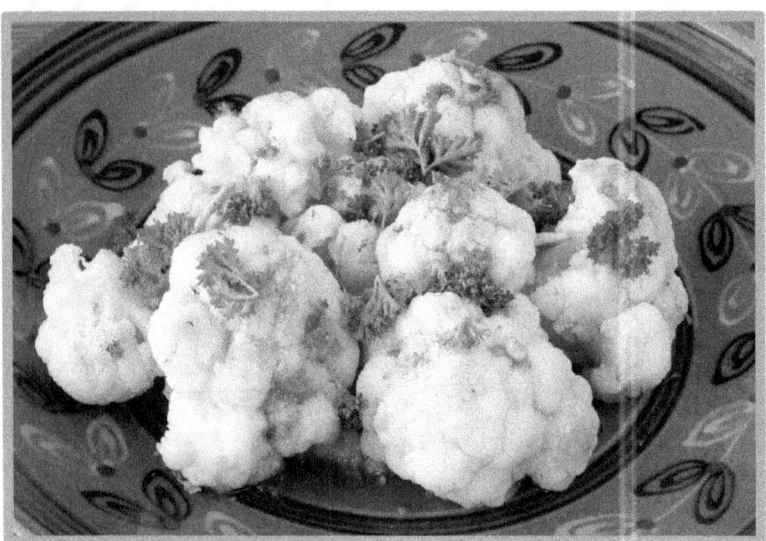

Servings: 2 to 3

Ingredients:

- 1 large head cauliflower
- 2 teaspoons curry powder
- ¼ cup olive oil
- Salt and pepper to taste

Instructions:

1. Preheat oven to 450°F and line a rimmed baking sheet with foil.
2. Cut the cauliflower into bite-size pieces and toss them in a mixing bowl with the curry powder, olive oil, salt and pepper.
3. Spread the cauliflower on the baking sheet and roast for 30 to 40 minutes until browned on the outside.
4. Let the cauliflower cool for 5 minutes before serving.

Chapter Four: After You Detox

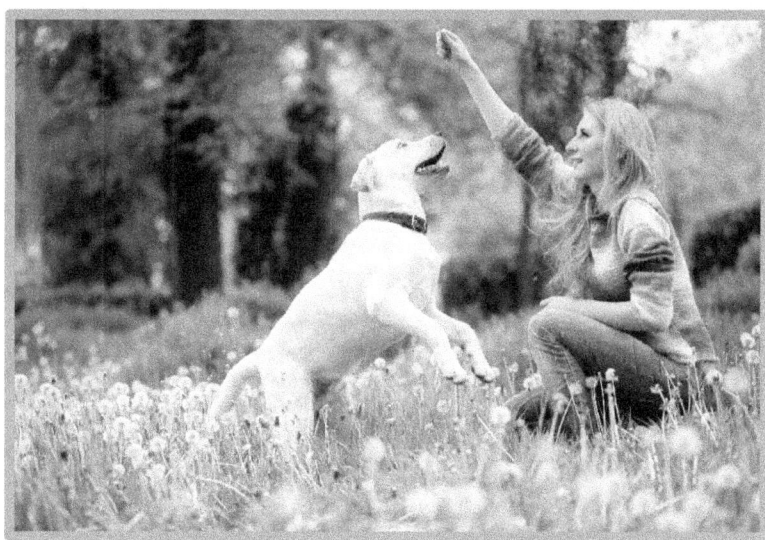

After you make it through the entire 21-day detox, you are faced with the decision of reintroducing sugar into your diet or keeping it out. This decision is entirely up to you and it should be made based on your personal preferences as well as your body's reaction to sugar. Some people have more severe reactions to the consumption of sugar and may do better if they continue to follow a completely sugar-free diet. Others may be able to tolerate small amounts of sugar – every case is different so it is your job to decide what is right for you.

If you decide to reintroduce sugar into your diet, start by adding small amounts of natural sugar – a handful of berries as a snack or a piece of fruit with lunch. As you reintroduce sugar, monitor your body's reaction to see how it affects you – if you have a bad reaction, you may want to continue to avoid sugar. However, if you do not experience any negative consequences then you can continue to add small amounts of natural sweeteners and, on occasion, refined sugars. The worst thing you can do up on finishing the sugar detox is to binge on sugary foods – this could put your body through an intense cycle of a sugar high followed by a crash.

Conclusion

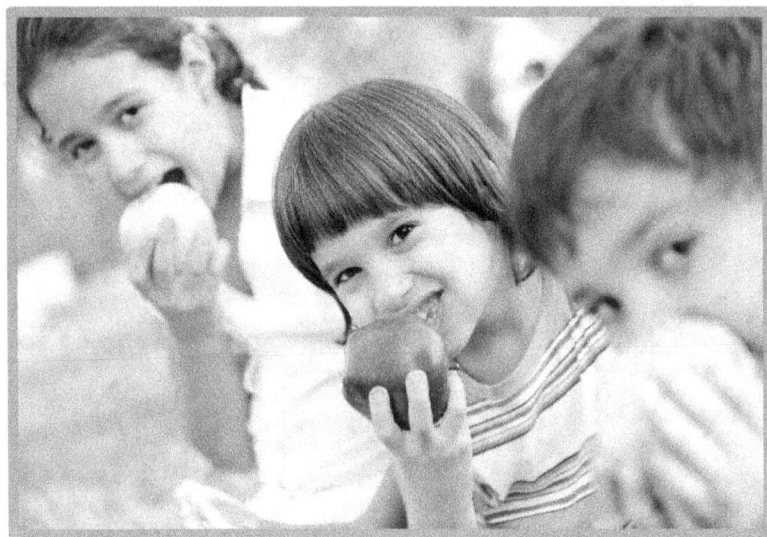

Hopefully after reading this book you have a better idea regarding what a sugar detox is and how it can benefit you. In reading this book you may have been shocked to discover just how much sugar you consume on a daily basis and what it may be doing to your body. Do not simply accept this information – you can make a simple change that will impact your health for the better. Consider engaging in a sugar detox yourself to break your sugar addiction and to kick cravings. If you are ready to rise to the challenge, you will find the recipes in this book are a great place to start.

What are you waiting for? Get started with your own Sugar Detox today!

www.ingramcontent.com/pod-product-compliance
Lightning Source LLC
Chambersburg PA
CBHW081751280526
45789CB00008B/2812